ON THE OTHER SIDE OF PAIN

HOW TO DISCOVER THE PURPOSE ON THE OTHER SIDE OF THE PAIN

VICKI HEAD JACKSON

ISBN 13: 978-0-9916687-9-3

For Worldwide Distribution, Printed in the U.S.A.

TABLE OF CONTENTS

DEDICATION

I dedicate this book to Gerald Jackson, my husband. This book is not only the result of my past; it is the result of your teachings. I am forever grateful for your support, prayers, and encouragement. It seems like yesterday we met and my life exploded in a sense, pertaining to the things of God. Your teaching has catapulted me to this new place. Thank you, man of Faith. Thank you, man of Wisdom. Thank you, man of God. I love you more than words can express.

ACKNOWLEDGEMENTS

First, let me thank my Lord JESUS Christ who has allowed this to be. I love Him with all of my heart, soul, and mind. He is the very reason that I live, move, and have my being.

Special thanks to our Pastors, Drs Mike and DeeDee Freeman. Thank you for your support, your believing in us, your love, your generosity, and most of all, life of Faith/a living example.

ON THE OTHER SIDE OF PAIN has been a journey that I did not believe could or would take place. There are many to thank, beginning with my husband Gerald, one of my biggest supporters, who made me believe in me and who taught me faith; if it's written, we can have it.

From the beginning of the process my oldest son, Dyterrius has been very encouraging, excited for me and very supportive. He is another big support.

I am grateful for my youngest son, Joshua. Thank you for coming every time I call. Joshua doesn't say a lot, but his support is just showing up. I love my boys.

To my brother, Carter, and his wife, Yvette, and my 2 sisters, Carnita and Letitia. I love you guys so much. I am the baby of the bunch and they all will go out of their way to help me in any way they can. I can call either one of them at any time for prayer and encouragement.

Thanks to my parents, Benjamin and Virginia, for all you instilled in me from the beginning. Thank you for taking the time to bring me up in church and rearing me in the admonition of The Lord. I am forever grateful to both of you. I am the product that you produced. I love you, mom and dad.

I have to give a shout out to my best friend, Annette, of 17 years. Thank you, Woman of God. You have been with me every step of the way; through blood, sweat, and tears. Thank you for praying without ceasing, for encouraging me and believing in me.

I also want to thank Elishia Dupree, my book coach/publisher/encourager of Write Way Publishing. I thank you and your staff for your expertise and encouragement.

Kingdom living ministries, I am honored to serve you and grateful for the love, thoughts, encouragement and intercession that has accompanied this process. Together, we are better.

INTRODUCTION

In the beginning, there was total chaos in my life. Let me share my story. I got married at age 19. After my mother told me not to. She said, "There's something about that man I don't like!" Well, to me, she just didn't want me to be happy. So I got married anyway. 2 months into the marriage, I found out that my husband had a child the same age as mine and that's when the abuse physical and verbal began. I was abused for several years without telling anyone. As a matter of fact, I made excuses for the black eyes and bumps and bruises saying that I had run into the wall or hit my head on the cabinet. He constantly cheated, even to the point of bringing the women in our home.

Did I fight back? Absolutely not! I was totally fearful of this man.

Out of a 7-day week, I would get beaten at least 2 of those days or more. If he was mad or had a fight with the other woman, I would have to pay; if he stayed out all night, I would have to pay; if he even thought that another man was looking at me, I would have to pay. The majority of the time he would be drunk. It was something about the alcohol that made him into this mad man. The abuse continued to happen, especially when he was drinking alcohol.

Finally, at the end of the 5th year, I had had all I could take, and in my mind, I knew if I stayed, I would eventually die. At that very moment, I chose life. My second son was 3 months old at the time and my oldest was 5.I packed our stuff and left what I called HELL. He was determined not to let go. He began to stalk me. I tried to get a restraining order against him and was unsuccessful; he raped me, kidnapped me, and threatened to kill me. In college at the time, he would even show up on the campus and harass me. I was going to church but that was all. I never had a personal relationship with God. You know, it was just the thing to do. I had become so tired of the fighting, the running and looking over my shoulders. I knew I needed help and no one in the natural would help me. I felt like this would end in my death if something didn't change.

One day, I woke up and decided to have a talk with this God that I heard about Sunday after Sunday. I began to cry out to Him and I said to Him, "This pain is too great for me; I need your help and if you are real, save me from this man or just let me die at his hand." It was so bad that I was choosing death over the situation. But GOD!!! All of a sudden, things started happening to him. Every time he would threaten me, on his way to do it, something would happen. It happened so much that he asked me, "What are you doing to me?" My response was, "I told my father, God, on you, so you better leave me alone. I am now protected from you." Ever since then, I never had another problem with him. The next time I saw him, we were in divorce court and a permanent restraining order was issued.

After all God had done, I continued to go to church, but again, it was just that. What I didn't realize is that I needed healing from the abuse. So my response to the pain was promiscuity. It was just a temporary fix. My life was a downward spiral. I thought I was the only woman messed up in that area. There was never a woman transparent enough to say, "I have dealt with that issue." So I thought I was all alone and too embarrassed to ask for help.

One night, I fell on my face on my kitchen floor. Here goes the same statement as before: "God, if you are real, please deliver me."

I don't believe that this is what I was created for; I don't believe that this is my only purpose for living, and if you don't deliver me from this promiscuity, then eventually I will die like this." I was not at the church. I was in my home alone because I did not think that the church could help.

The next morning, I woke up different. I knew something had changed about me. I looked in the mirror and said "Hi" to the new Vicki.

CHAPTER 1
THE CRUSHING

How did I get to this place? I imagine a life so different.

First, before I answer, God isn't the author of pain. The world he created was a world without pain, a paradise where the word suffering wasn't in the dictionary. The experience of relentless, unending pain was not designed by heaven; it invaded our lives from another agency. Let's look at Luke 13:10-17. The woman had a spirit of infirmity (a falling or defect in a person's character lacking power, disability). An evil spirit that oppresses people with spiritual, emotional or physical sickness (deception). Vs 16: "And ought not this woman, being a daughter of Abraham, whom Satan hath bound, lo these 18 years, be loosed from this bond of Satan." No, our pain doesn't come from God. True pain can turn out to be a blessing. It can even be a life saver. Pain ended up being a life saver for me.

DAY 1. 2 months into the marriage, I came home from work to confront my ex-husband about a phone call that I received. The person informed me that my ex-husband had a 3-month-old baby boy. I was crushed. I never would have thought that the man who said he loved me would have done this to me. We had been married for 2 months and our son was 9 months old. You do the math. They were only 7 months apart. Well, it did not go as planned. I thought that he would lie, beg, or say sorry. Instead, he began to beat me for finding out the truth about him. He slammed me to the floor and kicked me like a dog. So, in my mind, I was wondering, "What could I have done so bad that would cause this man to beat me as if he was fighting another man?" I felt bad for even confronting him. I had never experienced such rage. I was terrified. I never fought back because I was afraid for my life. From that day forward, I would get beat at least two times a week. I can remember this man spitting in my face and daring me to say anything. It was as if he hated me for no cause. I really felt that he was sent to destroy my life. There were times when women would call my home phone and ask to speak with him and I had to give him the phone or else he would beat me. He would sit in my face and talk to other women, and again, if I said something, I had to pay. I was terrified of this man. He totally disrespected me. I was treated like a roommate instead of a wife. For example, He had a heated fight with his so-called mistress, he came home so upset about it that he began to tell me about their problems. He went as far as telling me, "I am done with her; we broke up tonight." Now, maybe it's just me but there's something about this statement that just doesn't sound right to a wife.

I was crushed mentally, spiritually, and physically. I felt defeated, trapped, and confused. How could this be happening to me? I promised myself to never be with a man who is verbally or physically abusive. I can remember, as a child, watching my father abuse my mother. I can remember crying and shaking in fear and trying to get in between them. I watched this abuse for years. I would often say, as a child, "I will never let a man abuse me or cheat on me like my mom did." Unfortunately, I did the very thing that I said I wouldn't do; DOMESTIC VIOLENCE CAN HAPPEN TO ANYONE, YET THE PROBLEM IS OFTEN OVERLOOKED, EXCUSED, OR DENIED. Violence is not prejudice. In spite of size, gender, or race, many people have experienced it. Some people have died, but by the grace of God, I live to tell the rest of the story.

I experienced this abuse for 5 years. Every time I tried to leave, he would threaten to kill me, so I stayed. He would say, "If I can't have you, nobody will." He would say he loves me to death and he meant just that. The times that I got the courage to leave, he found me and threaten me so I would return home. I made excuses for the bruises and the black eyes—that I ran into the wall or hit my head on the cabinet. I blamed myself for the abuse; I felt responsible for his actions.

Everything seemed to be falling apart. I felt like I'd been punched into a bad dream. My life felt like a nightmare. It has been said, "Time heals all wounds." I do not agree. I've wasted time thinking things would get better. I've been crushed like grapes forced into olive oil. I was broken into tiny fracture pieces and unable to gain my strength. At this point, denying that he was abusive did not help. Every time I looked at my bruises, truth was staring me in the face. I then isolated myself from everyone including my love ones. I never told anyone in my family that I was being abused. They actually heard it in the streets. I can remember an incident in particular where my ex-husband and I had gone to the club. Well, he ended up getting together with another girl who was there at the club and told me to find a way home. So an old friend of my brother and his girlfriend ended up taking me home. Little did I know something happened with the girl that he was trying to get with. He got home before I did. In his mind, he is thinking that I must have gotten with another man. Oh, now that was a problem. Well, when the guy and his girlfriend got me to my house, I could not get in because he had something blocking the door. Then, out of nowhere, he came running towards me and knocked me down on the ground and began to beat me, thinking that I had been with another man because it took me too long to get home. This guy who was a friend of my brother just watched this man beat me and did absolutely nothing—oh, except tell other people, including my brother, what happened.

I later found myself bargaining with my ex-husband. Bargaining is the normal reaction to feelings of helplessness and vulnerability. I would say things like, "…If only we had sought counseling sooner…if only I had not addressed the things I knew about him…if only we had tried to be better persons towards each other." These thoughts only led to more depression and anger. I felt like I couldn't win for losing.

I began to blame myself for everything. In my mind, I felt like I was being punished for something, so I began to literally sit back and reminisce on my life to see what I could recall that could have caused all this.

I continued to stay and here we are past the fifth year. I am pregnant with our second child. Our oldest son was 4 years at the time. I worked a second shift job from 3-11pm. Well, for about a week, every night I got home from work, my son would say, "Mommy, I and dad were holding the baby." Of course, my ex-husband said that he was just a child and did not know what he was talking about. My son would not let it go, so now I knew that something wasn't right. A few days later, I began to talk with my father-in-law about what my son had told me. Something happened that I did not expect. He said, "Sit down let me talk to you because I am tired of this." Immediately, my heart began racing with uncertainty. He said, "Your husband has a newborn baby in Athens," and he and Dyterrius, my 4-year-old, have been driving there every day to see this baby.

Wow! Here goes the CRUSHING AGAIN. I think that was the most painful act of the entire relationship. I could not work that day. I just rode around screaming and crying. I confronted him about what I knew and again, just as the first time I found out about the 3-month-old baby, he began to beat me again for what I knew about him. By the way, this second baby and my second baby were 7 months apart as well. Now, this situation hit where it really hurts—my heart. This act began to really destroy my self-esteem. In my mind, if he will drive 2 hours every day to see a newborn, sign the birth certificate; ok, he really has to love this young lady. At the time, I was wondering, "What is wrong with me? Why has this man cheated and beat me the entire marriage? Am I not pretty enough? Maybe I'm too skinny." So once again, I felt like it was my fault. Could I be the reason for him cheating?

Studies show that 56% of men who have affairs claim to be happy in their marriages. It has been said that some men cheat because of low self-esteem. When a man is lacking self-esteem, he's more likely to enter martial affairs searching for significance. That's not a woman's fault. Usually, it's related to his insecurities.

After being sick and tired, I moved out for a couple of months. Then he showed up begging, saying how much he loved me and that he could not live without me. You know, the same stuff that they say. Well, I moved back mainly because I was pregnant at the time and did not want to do it alone. This was just another excuse to go back to the same old prison.

Later giving birth to my son, I can remember getting up through the night to care for him and my ex was never home. He constantly stayed the night away from home. I was very tired at this point. You know people can call you stupid, crazy, or tell you that you should leave but it's not until you get sick and tired yourself; then once your mind is made up, it's made up. My ex-husband had come home drunk after staying out all night and began to beat me because I confronted him. I will never forget looking up as he beat me; I could see my 5-year-old standing in a corner shaking in fear. I was reminded of myself as a little girl standing, shaking in fear as my dad beat my mom. That did it!! I began to talk out loud to myself and I said, "You may be ok with the cheating and the abuse, but don't make your child suffer." He was a musician in the church and this particular Sunday I decided not t go with him because I had already made up in my mind that I was leaving. This time, FOR GOOD!

Well, after he realized that I was really gone, things began to turn for the worst. He would sit at the edge of my mom's driveway and just watch the house all day. We called the police and they said that there was nothing they could do, because he was not on our property. He would stalk. It's so strange that I would never see him following me, but by the time I got to my destination, he showed up. I was attending Gordon College at the time and he would show up on the campus. Again, no one would help. He began threatening me, saying if I did not come back to him, he would kill me. Well, I knew for sure that if I went back, he would kill me, so not being with him, I felt I had a better chance of living.

Finally, I got tired of the threats and the stalking. I went to the court to get a restraining order and it was denied. They said that it was my word against his, and unless I had a witness, there was no proof of these accusations. I tried several times. I would call the police several times a week until they got tired of it. One day, I was hanging out with my friends and he came out of nowhere, snatched me up and walked away with me. People were watching and did nothing. He carried me to an apartment that was right around the corner from my mom's house. He had a gun and he raped me over and over. By night, I could hear the police siren and I knew that they were looking for me. They were knocking on the doors at this apartment complex. He said to me, "If the police knock on this door, I will kill you." I knew that God was with me because they never knocked on that door.

When he finally fell asleep I tried to leave quietly. But by the time I grabbed to the door knob, he grabbed me and took my clothes. I knew I was going to die and, really, at that point, I didn't care. I was just tired. The next morning, he woke up and said, "Get your clothes so that I can walk you home." I really didn't know how to receive that. I felt he would have me walk in front and shoot me in the back. He watched me walk home and did not harm me. I looked back and he was just standing, watching. I ran home. It was the grace of God all around me. When I got home, my mom called the police. He was arrested. The police said to me, "We have 3 charges against him—rape, stalking, and kidnapping." He was sure to do 7 years in prison. The officer said, "Please, don't take us through this if you are going to later drop the charges." Well, to say the truth, I dropped the charges.

CHAPTER 2
AN EMOTIONAL BASKET CASE

At this point my mind was so confused, I didn't know rather I was going or coming. The pain of my past affected me in more ways than I could imagine. It was extremely hurtful, I was very angry and bitter. I didn't understand why I had to go through what I went through. I began to ask in my mind, "What did I do to deserve this?" It was the worst thing I've ever experienced.

As you can see, family patterns are transferable. I adopted my mom's behavior as an enabler. Familiarity is a powerful magnet. It will draw people to re-create what they were taught, even if those lessons were unfulfilling or painful. I did my best to ignore the pain but it only got worse, I actually tried to move on and start over.

Starting over was a great decision; however, when I was alone, I still had to deal with me. I had to live with this broken person that I had become. I hated myself for allowing my emotions to rule my life. My emotions began to rule my life in such a way that I became hopeless and reckless. I was behaving in ways I thought I would never do. I became very loose and promiscuous.

I didn't like myself, I didn't love myself, I didn't think I had worth. I felt like I was ugly, that I was unattractive; all of this just made me feel less than a woman. I was just drained of everything that I thought I possessed. I was empty, I was confused, I was wounded, and I really couldn't share with anybody what I was experiencing because I really couldn't express it for myself. I felt very vengeful because of the many times my husband cheated on me. So what did I do? As the saying goes, "Hurting people hurt people." And that is so true. What I decided to do was, destroy other people's marriages. In my mind, I wanted revenge. So I began to hurt other people. I wanted other married women to feel the hurt that I felt. I wanted them to know what it felt like to see your husband grab hold of another woman, to embrace another woman, and to be with another woman. I wanted them to know what I felt like when my husband was bringing women into my home, when he was riding them in our car, when he was buying them gifts and not buying me gifts, respecting them and not respecting me. I wanted them to know how I felt, so my thing was, "I've got to get back at them." And at that particular time, because I couldn't think, I was thinking out of hurt, so my response to the situation was getting even.

Thus I began to hurt other people. It made me feel good for the moment because I began to say, "Now I'm not the only one." This went on for a while and I literally lost my identity. I had no clue of who I was anymore. I was brought up in the church as a little bitty girl singing in the choir and on the usher board, and wherever there was a need, I would do it. I loved to sing. I didn't have a personal relationship with God, but I was in church every Sunday and I had heard about this God, but for some reason, I could not even pull on that at the moment. I would still go to church but would leave church still broken, and still hurting, and still wounded and still wondering why this God they were talking about would allow this to happen to me. I had a lot of why's. There was a song they used to sing at the church and the song was, "I don't know why I have to cry sometimes; I don't know why I have to suffer sometimes." This song resonated in my spirit, and every day, I thought about this song. So I began to verbally say, "I don't know why I had to go through this; I don't know why I had to suffer." And because I was having an identity crisis, I was even saying, "I don't even know who

I am; I don't even know to whom I belong." I felt all alone; I felt like I was in a world all by myself. And I felt like I was the target of hurt. I was very, very bitter and angry at everybody.

The thing is, this same man moved on with this life and got into other relationships and there I was; I could not find a serious relationship because I just wanted to hurt somebody for what he had done to me. I didn't understand how he seemed to be happy after all the hell he had put me through. I didn't think it was fair. Sadly, this went on for about four years—me just dealing with the hurt, me being promiscuous, and feeling like I'm out to hurt somebody.

In spite of all this, I still kept going to church; there was still something inside that kept me moving toward the things of God. Every time I heard the Word of God preached, something would resonate inside my spirit. I could hear the Holy-Spirit reminding me, "This is not who you are." So, all of a sudden, it seems like I began to recognize that this is not who I am, I've got to be better than this, I've got to live better than this, I've got to do better than this and that all the promiscuity was just too much for me. There was a void there that I was trying to fill with sex.

My emotions were steering out of control but I didn't know how to stop these destructive behaviors. Having sex with other men was my way of receiving the love I was missing. Unfortunately, the void was still there. I was expecting someone to address my issue but no one was transparent enough to talk about those issues. The women in my church were too sanctified to mention worldly matters. Everyone would have their hats and their suits, and they would quote all these scriptures and would just walk and talk the talk, but nobody said that they had any problems. So here I am again, all alone. Me and my issues, me and my hurt, and my pain, my anger and my bitterness, and destroying my life with my lifestyle.

One day while I was in my house, I will never forget it, I fell on my kitchen floor, and there I was with the same statement that I had already given God twice—I said, "God, if you are real, you will take this from me." I began to cry and I said, "God, I know you did not create me for promiscuity; I know you did not create me for this; I know you did not create me to go through hurt all of my life; I know you did not create me to go through pain for the rest of my life; I know you did not create me to get beat, to get cursed out, to get abused, to get cheated and trampled on. I know you did not create me for this. I don't know what you created me for, but I know it can't be this. So if you don't take this promiscuity from me, I'm going to die just like this." But I wanted to live and I said it over and over again, "God, I want to live, and if you love me, and you are real, I need you to deliver me today." I actually fell asleep in my kitchen on the floor and when I woke up, I felt different; there was something different about me. I looked in the mirror and to me, I didn't even look the same, and I literally said "Hi" to the new Vicki. And from that point on, I began to gather myself. I began to get involved with God and the Church for real.

October 1996, I gave my life to God and said, "God, I want you to save me from sin, from the ugly way of living, from this nasty, bitter lifestyle, and I want you to help me forgive those who hurt me so that I can move forward in the things of God. So I began to really live this thing for God. The promiscuity ceased immediately and I knew then that this God that I had been hearing about, that I had been hearing people preach about for years, I found out for myself that He's real. I'm reminded of a scripture that says, "Come as you who are heavy laden and burden and I will give you rest. Take this yoke upon you, learn of me, for my yoke is easy, and my burdens are light." I begin to hear that over and over in my mind and I just began to declare that. Every day, I found myself getting stronger and I was getting better.

> You know, I felt like the woman with the issue of blood; she had been with that thing for all of those years, oh Jesus! And there was nobody that could help her. She went from doctor to doctor and that void was not filled—she was still bleeding. And that's how I was; I went from one man to the other trying to get that void filled, but I was left still bleeding, still wondering what's next, who's next. But I finally got to Jesus; and the Bible says that she pressed her way through the crowd. And I just believe that as she pressed her way, there were some people that knew her situation and did not want to get close to her because she had been bleeding for so long. I believe she had an odor, and I believe as she pressed her way through the crowd, people were pushing her out of the way, talking about her, laughing at her. The same thing with me; I believe in this situation, in this promiscuity, in this lifestyle that I developed through hurt and pain, that people were talking about me. As I was trying to make my way to Jesus, I know that there were some people laughing at me because my husband cheated, because he beat me; there were some women who talked about me. They said, "Evidently, she can't satisfy her husband." To them, it was a game. But I kept trying to get to Jesus. I said, "I'm going to get there if it's the last thing I do because He is the only doctor that is left that can help me." So, just like the woman with the issue of blood; when she got to Jesus, she touched the hem of His garment and what she

> wanted was so real that it pulled something from Him. He knew someone had touched him in the crowd. That's how I was when I got to Jesus. I begin to hold on to him for dear life because I knew my very life depended on me getting to Jesus. And when I got to him, I held on and I held on for a long time.

In 1999, I was filled with the Holy Ghost. In January of 2000, I announced to the church that God had called me to preach the gospel of Jesus Christ, and in April of 2000, I did my very first sermon and the name of that sermon was "I won't go back." Oh, Jesus! You see, to them, it is was just a sermon, but this was my declaration to the Lord. Because of where I had come from, I knew I had been delivered; I knew the hand of God had touched my life; I knew it and that was my declaration. Even today, "I won't go back." So I went on and I preached; this was in 2000. Now I'm preaching the gospel, traveling to places, people being healed, people being delivered, people being set free. One thing about me is I decided to be transparent. I remember when I was in my mess, I never heard a woman of God tell the truth, what she was going through, what she battled with, or what she dealt with in her flesh, so I felt I was all alone. For this reason, I told God I would be transparent; I want to let the world know, I want to let hurting women know where I came from, where I had been and where I am right now. So I began to tell my story in different places because I wanted people to know that God is a deliverer, He is still healing, He is still setting free. Because the very thing I thought God could not do, He did for me and I am forever grateful.

After years of fulfilling the call of God on my life, I was believing God for a husband—I mean I was single from 1992 to 2008, loving God, spending time with God, celebrating God. I had a singles ministry teaching women how to be single, how to be content in singleness. But at the time, I was lonely; I believed I needed a man of God. So I kept believing God for a husband and so many people began to prophecy to me "Oh, you are going to have a husband by the end of the year" and that year went by, and another year went by. I began to get discouraged. But when I least expected, though I knew what I had asked God for, I was in a place, and I walked into this store. When I walked into this store, this gentleman and I made eye contact, and immediately, I felt I heard the Lord say, "This is your husband." As soon as I heard that, the gentleman walked up to me and said, "God told me that you are my wife." Now let me just put a pin in that real quick, because I want to go ahead and get some things clear; so many times we go around and we say things like "God said this is my husband"; "God said this is my wife"; well, in the garden, when God made Eve, Adam was the one that said, "This is bone of my bone, and flesh of my flesh"; He never said to Adam, "This is your wife." What we have to understand about God is, if He says, "This is your husband"; "This is your wife," there is no failure in God. So if your marriage fails, then that couldn't have been God. What God will do is that He will present that thing before you; but He made us free moral will agents, so He will present it before you, but you have a chose. The Bible declares, "A man that finds a wife finds a good thing and obtains favor from the Lord." It did not say, "God that finds a wife." Even after we get married, we expect God to keep our marriage. Well, listen, God ordains marriage; He won't keep your marriage. Why? I am glad you asked. He has given us in His Holy word, writings of men and women inspired by God, teachings and training manuals to help lead, guide and instruct us.

CHAPTER 3
SPIRITUAL PARALYSIS

And so I said, "I know that this is God; this is my husband because GOD said it."

I married this man without trying to find out anything. I just knew it was God, and within seven days, we were married. Well, everything was cute at first. Six months into the marriage, he didn't come home and when he did, we began to talk; now he did tell me from the beginning that he had had an addiction to drugs in the past, but he said that he had been delivered for fifteen years or better so; of course I believe that because I know God had delivered me; I believed God could deliver anybody from anything, so that didn't matter to me. So here we are six months into the marriage and this man comes home the next day saying, "I'm sorry but I fell," and me being who I am, the spiritual woman of God, I said, "It's okay." So I kind of patted him and said, "It's okay; we are going to get through this, we are going to pray you through this." Now at this point, I was thinking, "I am so spiritual, I am so Holy Ghost filled and so fire baptized, and speaking in tongues, and laying on my face and fasting." I thought that I could deliver him. Well, how many of us know that God is the deliverer? Hallelujah.

So six months later, here comes another fall. Again, we were going to pray through this; I didn't get mad about it. So here we are six months later; okay, now the spiritual girl had sat down, the old girl had stood up and she's mad, angry, and bitter. So now I'm trying to figure out, "What am I going to do with you?" Of course he cried and he begged; he said, "I know God is going to do this, and we are going to walk through this together." At this point, I had told everybody that this was God; now, I'm embarrassed to let anybody know it wasn't God. This was a decision I made in my flesh and I'm going to have to deal with the consequences.

At that point, I packed my stuff and I left to start a new life. I got another place and I started over. But when I got to this place, my growth became stunted—because of the pain, and because of the paralysis. So even though I was out of that addiction situation, I was still paralyzed because the hurt now became magnified, the bitterness was magnified, the anger was really, really magnified. I was so angry with this man for destroying my life that I wanted harm to come to him; oh yes, miss sanctified, miss Holy Ghost filled, fire baptized. I wanted him to suffer, I wanted him to pay for what I was going through. I wanted him to feel the embarrassment, so I begin to trash him, I begin to tell everybody that he was on crack, he was nothing, he's going to be on the streets, he's going to lose everything. That wasn't the character of God, but I was paralyzed; I couldn't walk in the things of God at that moment. I went into a serious, serious depression. I locked my doors, I didn't answer my phone, I didn't want to talk to anybody, I didn't want to go to church, I didn't want to pray, I didn't want to read my Bible. I literary felt paralyzed.

I had no energy and I had heard a lot of people talk about depression and how they were suicidal and I thought it was stupid. I thought it was the craziest thing I had ever heard until it hit me. Now here I am sitting in my bathtub and the devil is saying, "You can go ahead and take your life and all of those that are not here to help you; you can make them feel guilty." That sounded real good to me at that moment because I was saying, "I have been there for everybody. Every time somebody was sick, I was there; every time somebody was depressed, I was there; every time somebody was suicidal, I was there; every time somebody needed money, if I had it, I was there; every time somebody was on the street and didn't have anywhere to live, I was there." So I felt, "Here I am in a situation all alone, all by myself, not going to church and no one is even checking on me. How dare they not help me?" I became even more bitter with the church.

Paralysis is the loss of muscle movement in the body. Our sense of movement is controlled by communication between the sensory nerves (which are part of the peripheral nervous system) and the central nervous system (comprised of the brain and spinal cord). Disruption of communication of nerve impulses anywhere along the pathway from the brain to the muscles can impair control of muscle movement and cause muscle weakness and loss of coordination. Muscle weakness can progress to paralysis, loss of the ability to move the muscles.

Paralysis symptoms can occur anywhere in the body. They may occur on both sides of the body (bilateral) or one side (unilateral). I was weak, dysfunctional and stressed out.

One day, in the midst of all this, I was sitting in my office at work. It was the end of the day and I was the only one left at the office trying to catch up. All of a sudden, my thoughts were not coming together; I felt like I was in a whirlwind. My hands were shaking and I felt very nervous and scared. All I knew to do was to call my best friend, Annette, and my exact words were, "Help me; I feel like I am losing my mind." Immediately, I began to pray and I started to feel better at that moment. I prayed until I was totally free from the attacks on my mind. During this spiritual paralysis, I almost lost my mind. I almost had a breakdown. So now when I say, "I THANK GOD FOR MY MIND," is it just a cliche or something cute to say? NO, I REALLY THANK GOD FOR MY MIND. There are some people who went through what I went through, and ended up in a mental facility.

One rainy evening, I was at home and there was a knock on the door; it was some people from my church. I was pastoring a flock but I had actually shut the church down and we were going to another church because I could not do it—I could not continue to hurt the people, because I was preaching out of hurt; I was wounded, I was broken and if I could just tell the truth about where I was, I could not help them. I loved them so much that I needed them to get the help that they needed. So I gathered them up and I said, "Let's go here and sit in this ministry until I'm restored." I took them to this ministry and then I just stopped going because I couldn't go anymore; I didn't want to go anymore, I didn't even want to talk to anyone. So these people showed up at my house and when they came, what I expected to happen didn't happen. I expected them to come in and pray and encourage me and say, "Get up and get on your feet." No; instead, they said to me, "Why are you like this? We need you. You can't be down; we need you." Well, to me, that was selfish. They were thinking about themselves; they were thinking about what I could do for them, and with that, I even became angrier at the church. Needless to say, by the time they left my house, I was worse off than I was before they got there. And I'm not blaming them; I don't think they knew what to do or what to say. So I was grateful that they even tried, that they even attempted to do something, but what they brought was not what I needed. That was a learning experience for me, because a lot of times when people are in situations, even in death situations, we walk in as preacher and pastors and teachers and we say the wrong things. So I learned in that state that all I needed was somebody there. Don't talk to me; just be there.

A few days after that, my armorbearer at the time came to my house; she came in through the door and said, "Hi, pastor!" She sat down on my floor and watched television. She never said another word to me. That was the best day that I had had in a long time. All I needed was for somebody to be in my presence. And what I have learned from that is "Just shut your mouth and be there."

A couple of days later, I was still down and a few months later—well, it was a year later—I just said, "You know what? I just need a new start." I really felt that I was led of the Lord to just start over, and I needed to just get away and deal with me. I relocated to Tampa, Florida. When I got to Tampa and it was very, very scary; I was very fearful of the unknown. I felt it was the right thing to do but at the same time, it was the unknown that I was very fearful of.

I was sitting in my new apartment with no one but me. Negative thoughts kept flowing through my head. I was disappointed about all the bad decisions I'd made. I had a lot of unanswered questions and too many open doors. If I could fix this situation I would do it in a heartbeat. I wanted to scream.

As I began to work, I began to meet people and that helped a lot because my job was my outlet and that was where I wanted to be all the time, I avoided being alone to deal with my inner conflict. My mother, best friends, Annette and Montez, and my sister Carnitia were supportive ears during this difficult season. If it weren't for them, I would be like a ship without a sail.

And so, I was still at a point where I felt stagnated. I wasn't sure why I wasn't able to move in the things of God freely. Saved but still hurting with a whole lot of issues. Although I was in a new city and I had a fresh start, I was still broken. I relapsed. And those that understand addiction, there are triggers that come that will cause you to relapse. You can be doing well for one minute then all of a sudden there goes a setback. This is a prime example of unmet needs, unhealed hurts, and unresolved issues. The pain is like an open cut that we refuse to treat. If we don't deal with an open cut it will become infected. You see, one thing about a cut: after so many hours, you can't stitch it up, because what you are doing is stitching up the infection. And I think that is what is happening with us in the body of Christ and even the people of the world; when we get hurt real bad and people really cut us we need to deal with the pain immediately within the boundaries of wise counsel. If we continue to shout over the pain, we will become infected and harder to reach. This is a great example of stitching up a wound that has been opened for too long and now there is an infection on the inside, and eventually, that infection is going to poison your whole bloodstream.

So here I am now; I've got to deal with this thing, but I don't know how to deal with it. Anyway, I actually went into this moment of not doing anything, but what happened? You see, God is so awesome; He just kind of divinely sets things in place and what I love about God is He gives us the choice, He presents these things to us, but it's our choice whether we receive it or not.

So what happened? I was in a drought, and one day I was headed back to Atlanta for the weekend and I stopped at this store, the name of the store was Victory-land and while I was in line at the store, there was a gentleman in line behind me—which is now my husband—and there was a lady in front of me, and I began to talk to the lady and I was telling her that I was getting ready to drive to Atlanta but it looked like it going to rain; he said to me, "Oh, it's not going to rain; the weather is going to be good today." So in my mind, I was thinking, "I am not talking to you; you don't want to deal with me; I have been in the gutter and back and now is not the time." But he continued to talk; we began to have a conversation, and when I got outside of the store, we continued to talk. We exchanged phone numbers and he asked me if I had a church, and he invited me to his church.

When I got back home, all of a sudden, I went back to reading my word; I went back to praying and fasting—and I mean…it was an immediate thing. And I can remember making the statement when I got home saying, "Who is this man?" And I pondered on that because, at the time, I could not understand what had transpired. And when I did the chapter on purpose, I touched on this "how purpose met purpose" and when I met him, the purpose that was on the inside of me connected with the purpose that was on the inside of him.

Just like when Mary went to Elizabeth and the baby leaped, purpose met purpose. So that's what happened, but remember, now I stitched up an opened wound that had been opened for a long time. Still, deliverance had not taken place; still, the healing was not complete. But I didn't understand it at the time, that's why I'm here to help you. So we had dates, and we prayed together and studied the word of God together and everything was going well. He proposed and I was like, "This is it! And this is an awesome man of God; we are growing together, we are reading together, we are studying together, we are fasting together." We both knew that there was a call on our lives to the nation. We knew that God had called us to transform lives—we knew this. So we got married—beautiful wedding ceremony; everything good. He even told me later that when he got home, he went back to the things of God because he was dealing with a lot of hurts as well. There were a lot of things that happened in his life that pushed him away from the things of God as well. So we were both hurting. All of a sudden, we were so spiritual and working and doing the things of God that we forgot we had not healed.

CHAPTER 4
PAIN

Even though I'm in a fresh new marriage, I still had unresolved pain. Pain—an unpleasant sensory and emotional experience associated with actual or potential feelings. The feelings are conveyed to the brain by sensory neurons. This discomfort signals actual or potential injury to the body.

SPIRITUAL DEFINITION—Spiritual distress and spiritual crisis occur when a person is unable to find sources of meaning, hope, love, peace, comfort, strength and connection in life or when conflict occurs between their beliefs and what is happening in their life. Spiritually speaking, pain has benefits:

1. One of the benefits of pain is expressed by JAMES 1: 2-3, *"CONSIDER IT ALL JOY, MY BRETHREN WHEN YOU ENCOUNTER VARIOUS TRIALS, KNOWING THAT THE TESTING OF YOUR FAITH PRODUCES ENDURANCE."*

According to James, when we endure trials, knowing that God is at work in us helps to produce endurance and Christ-like character. This applies to mental, emotional, and spiritual pain as well as physical.

2. Pain provides an opportunity to experience the grace of God. Consider, Paul, 2 COR 12: 9, *"AND HE HAS SAID TO ME, MY GRACE IS SUFFICIENT FOR YOU, FOR MY POWER IS PERFECTED IN WEAKNESS. MOST GLADLY, THEREFORE, I WILL RATHER BOAST ABOUT MY WEAKNESSES SO THAT THE POWER OF CHRIST MAY DWELL IN ME."*

Paul was speaking of a thorn in his flesh that was troubling him. We don't know what it was but it seemed to have been painful for Paul. He recognized that God's grace was being given to him, so he could endure. God will give his children the grace to bear the pain.

When we are in pain, it is an excellent time to realize that Jesus endured excruciating, emotional, and physical pain on our behalf.
** Know this, there is no pain that could compare to the horrific events of Jesus's Crucifixion, and he suffered that pain willingly to redeem us and to glorify HIS Father.

3. PAIN REFINES US.
ISAIAH 48: 10 *"BEHOLD, I HAVE REFINED THEE, BUT NOT WITH SILVER; I HAVE CHOSEN THE IN THE FURNACE OF AFFLICTION."*
pain has a way of bringing our strengths and weakness to the surface. When the dross (something regarded as worthless, rubbish, scum formed on the surface) floats to the surface, God skims it off; He purifies and refine us to be the radiant Bride of Christ.

4. PAIN PRODUCES GROWTH AND MATURITY
JAMES 1: 2-4 *"MY BROTHER COUNT IT ALL JOY WHEN YE FALL INTO DIVERS TEMPTATIONS, KNOWING THIS, THAT THE TRYING OF YOUR FAITH WORKETH PATIENCE."*
WHEN WE TURN TOWARD GOD IN OUR PAIN; HE CAN USE OUR SUFFERING TO MATURE OUR FAITH.

5. PAIN/SUFFERING CONFORMS US INTO THE IMAGE OF GOD.
ROM 8:28-29 *"AND WE KNOW THAT ALL THINGS WORK TOGETHER FOR GOOD TO THEM THAT LOVE GOD, TO THEM WHO ARE CALLED ACCORDING TO HIS PURPOSE. Vs. 29, FOR WHOM HE DID FOREKNOW,*

HE ALSO PREDESTINATE TO BE CONFORMED TO THE IMAGE OF HIS SON, THAT HE MIGHT BE THE FIRSTBORN AMONG MANY BRETHREN."

IF WE ARE WILLING TO SIT STILL AND LET GOD WORK, WE WILL FIND OURSELVES BEING TRANSFORMED INTO THE IMAGE OF JESUS. WHEN WE SEEK GOD THROUGH HIS WORD AND PRAYER, WE FIND JESUS. REMEMBER JESUS UNDERSTANDS OUR PAIN BECAUSE HE, TOO, SUFFERED.

I never looked at pain as a powerful tool until after so many failed attempts of trying to face pain alone. Now I understand how pain produces the Glory in our lives. It lets me know that pain has the power to push us into purpose or cause us to abort our purpose. Pain is really like a coming attraction that everyone anticipated coming—the preview before the real movie...The devil already had seen the movie and he doesn't want me to walk in it...Pain, if not handled properly, can cause delay or an abortion in God's plan for us…Pain causes us to call on God when he is nowhere in our plans, so pain is powerful. God loves us so much that he allows pain to get our attention so we won't go to sleep before the movie starts…

Let's scripturally deal with the powerless enemy with the power of God.

THE ENEMY IS POWERLESS. HE ONLY HAS THE POWER YOU GIVE HIM. EZEKIEL 28:13 *"THOU HAST BEEN IN EDEN THE GARDEN OF GOD; EVERY PRECIOUS STONE WAS THY COVERING, THE SARDIS TOPAZ, AND THE DIAMOND, THE BERYL, THE ONYX, AND THE JASPER, THE SAPPHIRE, THE EMERALD, AND THE CARBUNCLE AND GOLD; THE WORKMANSHIP OF THY TABRETS AND of THY PIPES WAS PREPARED IN THEE IN THE DAY THAT THOU WAST*

CREATED." SATAN WAS NOT SELF-EXISTENT LIKE GOD. HE IS A CREATED BEING.

LUKE 4:8 *"AND JESUS SAID UNTO HIM; GET THEE BEHIND ME SATAN, FOR IT IS WRITTEN, THOU SHALT WORSHIP THE LORD THY GOD AND HIM ONLY SHALT THOU SERVE."*

EPHESIAN 6:11 *"PUT ON THE WHOLE AMOUR OF GOD THAT YE MAY BE ABLE TO STAND AGAINST THE WILES OF THE DEVIL."*
WILES, DECEPTION, TRICKERY, DEVIOUS, CUNNING. HE HAS DECEPTION, NOT POWER.

REVELATION 12:9 *"AND THE GREAT DRAGON WAS CAST OUT, THAT OLD SERPENT, CALLED THE DEVIL AND SATAN, WHICH DECEIVETH*
THE WHOLE WORLD, HE WAS CAST OUT INTO THE EARTH AND HIS ANGELS WERE CAST OUT WITH HIM."
THE DECEIVER WAS STRIPPED OF HIS POWER AND ONLY LEFT WITH DECEIT.

MATTHEW 28:18 *"THEN JESUS CAME TO THEM AND SAID, 'ALL AUTHORITY IN HEAVEN AND ON EARTH HAS BEEN GIVEN TO ME.'"*

LUKE 10:18-19. *"JESUS REPLIED, I BEHELD SATAN FALL LIKE LIGHTNING FROM HEAVEN. VS. 19. BEHOLD, I GIVE YOU POWER TO TREAD ON SERPENTS AND SCORPIONS, AND OVER ALL THE POWER OF THE ENEMY AND NOTHING SHALL BY ANY MEANS HURT YOU."*

JESUS CLEARLY EXPLAINS IN JOHN 10: 10 *THAT THERE IS A THIEF OUT THERE IN THE DARKNESS. SOMEONE WHO WANTS TO KILL AND TO DESTROY AND BRING PAIN, BUT THEN HE ADDS THIS: "I AM COME THAT THEY MIGHT HAVE LIFE AND THAT THEY MIGHT HAVE IT MORE ABUNDANTLY."*

This is your season to be loosed from that thing that has had you bound. This woman had a disability, a pain, a condition. In the natural, she was getting worse. She did not think it could get better. Come on; let's look at this situation. You have been in your situation for too long and it seems that the pain is growing worse. Well, you are actually in a good place, believe it or not.

When this woman thought that all hope was gone, Jesus called her out from among the crowd. I believe in my sanctified mind that she was not the only one in the place with pain or an infirmity, but she was the one that He called out.

This pain or hurt that you are dealing with is just a tool to connect you with the real Jesus. See, you have been in the back too long. This is your coming out season. God is using that thing that has had you bound for so long to bring you to the Front. He will use your situation to put you before great men.

God has used my husband and I to be a support system for each other. We both realized that we were still hurt in some areas. Instead of running away from the marriage we ran to God. We have learned to be patient with one another and deal with our issues as they surface. During this process of your pain being displayed, it is important to have someone who's willing to love you through all your imperfections. Your true purpose is on the other side of this pain. Don't give up but keep pressing forward You are loosed of that pain. In Jesus name. You are walking through the pain now but Purpose is on the other end.

CHAPTER 5
PURPOSE

"The purpose of life is not to be happy. It is to be useful, to be honorable, to be compassionate, to have it make some difference that you have lived and lived well."

— Ralph Waldo Emerson

What is Purpose?

Purpose according to the Bible:
The purpose of life is goodness which God has prepared, according to Ephesians 2:10, "For we are His workmanship, created in Christ Jesus for good works, which God prepared beforehand that we should walk in them."

We are God's workmanship, created in Christ Jesus unto good works, which God hath before ordained that we should walk in them. We were created do good and to be partakers in the goodness which GOD has prepared. Life given by God is very valuable and should be used in accordance with the intent of our Creator.

How do you discover your real purpose in life?

I'm not talking about your job, your daily responsibilities, or even your long-term goals. I mean the real reason why you're here at all—the very reason you exist.

Perhaps you're a person who doesn't believe you have a purpose and that life has no meaning. Doesn't matter. Not believing that you have a purpose won't prevent you from discovering it. All that a lack of belief will do is make it a longer process. Most likely, though, if you don't believe you have a purpose, then you will continue to sit idle whiling away or not fulfilling why you came to this earth. You do have a purpose.

If you want to discover your true purpose in life, you must first empty your mind of all the false purposes you've been taught (including the idea that you may have no purpose at all).

So, how to discover your purpose in life? Let me give you a quick exercise.

Get out a sheet of paper,

Write at the top, "What is my purpose in life?"

Write the first answer that comes to mind.

Meditate on it for a moment. It should be the very thing that you are passionate about, you love doing, and you love it so much that you will do without pay. What words came to your mind? It should have brought tears to your eyes. This is your purpose.

That's it. Whatever you wrote may seem impossible or even silly, but it's okay. Recognizing what it is you were put on earth to do is the first step.

You may also discover a few answers that seem to give you a mini-surge of emotion, but they don't quite make you cry—they're just a bit off. Highlight those answers as you go along, so you can come back to them to generate new permutations. Each reflects a piece of your purpose, but individually, they aren't complete. When you start getting these kinds of answers, it just means you're getting warm.

Take a 2-minute break; close your eyes, relax, clear your mind, and focus on the intention for the answer to come to you—this is helpful as the answers you received will begin to have greater clarity.

When you find your own unique answer to the question of why you're here, you will feel it resonate with you deeply. The words will seem to bring a special energy to you, and you will feel that energy whenever you read them.

Discovering your purpose is the easy part. The hard part is keeping it with you on a daily basis and working on yourself to make it come to pass.

You have to get around positive people to help you to bring purpose to pass. I tell people all the time, "GET AWAY FROM THOSE WITH YOUR SAME PROBLEM AND GET WITH THOSE WHO HAVE YOUR SOLUTION."

The late Dr. Myles Munroe stated, "The graveyard is the richest place on earth." Why? Because so many people die without ever fulfilling their purpose. There are millionaire potentials in the grave; there are doctors who never moved towards their purpose; there are preachers who could have had worldwide ministries. Who hindered them? Or did they just not believe in themselves? Die empty with your purpose fulfilled.

Listen, I don't care what the devil has told you; I don't care how you feel, how things look or even what negative people have said to you. You were created with a purpose. There is a king in you. Find out what it is and walk in it.

You've got to get mad enough about where you are and do something about it.

I decree and declare that today marks a new starting point for you to believe, receive and, start walking in your purpose. I see you getting up out of that seat of doing nothing and switching to the next chair of doing something.

Luke 1:26-30.

This is the only scriptural reference that even suggests that Mary might be worthy of worship. The angel gives Mary a number of high compliments; still, nothing indicates that she is worthy of worship, sinless for her entire life, or given any other honor aside from being God's chosen vessel for the purpose of the Son of God being made flesh and blood. This is truly a great honor, but God has throughout the ages chosen various people to fulfill different roles according to His will and purpose—and none of them are shown to be worthy of worship.

So it doesn't matter what you feel about you or what people feel about you. There is a God-ordained purpose to be fulfilled.

In verse 28, Angel Gabriel tells Mary in his salutation that she is "highly favored," and in verse 30, that she "has found favor with God." The Greek word translated highly favored to mean "grace," "to endure with special honor," or "to be accepted." From this example, we can see that being "highly favored" is not synonymous with being worthy of worship. Everyone in the body of Christ is highly favored because God has accepted us through the justification brought about by Christ's sacrifice.

In verse 30, Angel Gabriel tells Mary that she has found favor with God. "Favor" is the Greek word Charis, which means "graciousness of manner or action." This notes favor on the part of the giver and thankfulness on the part of the receiver. Gabriel tells Mary that she is the chosen one, of grace and favor by God—the emphasis is on what God is doing. We see nothing in this verse to give any indication that Mary should be worshipped. She simply received God's favor by being chosen to fulfill this role or purpose.

Vs 31: "You will conceive and give birth to a son, and you are to call him JESUS." What we can conceive, we can achieve Vs 34: "'How will this be,' Mary asked the angel, 'since I am a virgin.'"
Let's deal with this.

vir•gin
—a person who has never had sexual intercourse;
a person who is naive, innocent, or inexperienced, especially in a particular context:
not yet touched, used, or exploited:
untouched, unspoiled, untainted, immaculate, pristine, ...

God is looking for virgins. Can he use you? He is looking for those who haven't done it yet. See, this purpose that God is bringing forth in you is new; you have never done this before; it's untouched, untainted. So I'm glad that you are a virgin and you have no clue of how to do this thing called purpose. God does not need your expertise; we just need His.

There are two elements needed to bring purpose alive.
1. The Holy Spirit
2. Elizabeth

Vs 35, 36: "The angel answered, 'The Holy Spirit will come upon you and the power of the most high will overshadow you. So the holy one to be born will be called the son of God.

Even Elizabeth, your relative, is going to have a child in her old age, and she who was said to be unable to conceive in her sixth month."

See, this thing is so big that the Holy Spirit has to get involved to bring it to pass. Elizabeth is that person who has already been through the morning sickness; the pain, the anguish of the first trimester.

As earlier mentioned, we need to get away from those with our problem and get with those who have our solution. You are a product of who you hang around. If you are in poverty and accompany poverty, guess what------- You can fill in the blank.

Because Elizabeth is ahead of you in this birthing of purpose, then she can assist and encourage you through your pain. See, you don't understand what takes place yet because you were just impregnated with purpose but Elizabeth has the answers to encourage you when you want to quit, give up or just throw in the whole towel. I believe she can share with you the scriptures that held her together when she wanted to quit.

You: "This labor pain is too much to bear."

Elizabeth: "Be ye steadfast, unmovable always abounding in the work of The Lord, knowing that your labor is not in vain."

You: "The affliction is too much."

Elizabeth: "Many are the afflictions of the righteous but He shall deliver us out of them all."

You: "This seems and looks impossible."

Elizabeth: "With God, all things are possible" (Matt 9:29).

You: "I feel so weak, I have no more strength to fight."

Elizabeth: "And He said unto me, 'My grace is sufficient for thee; for my strength is made perfect in weakness" (2 Cor. 12:9-11).

You: "It feels as if everyone is against me."

Elizabeth: "What shall we then say to these things? If God be or us, who can be against us?"

Vs 39-41: "At that time Mary got ready and hurried to a town in the hill country of JUDEA where she entered Zechariah's home and greeted Elizabeth.

When Elizabeth heard Mary's greeting, the baby leaped in her womb, and Elizabeth was filled with the Holy Spirit."

Purpose met purpose. Earlier, I shared how I was in a dead place in my life. I felt defeated. But regardless of how you feel, purpose is still present. Well, I met my husband, and immediately, something happened that I did not understand at the time. All I know is that I didn't feel like reading, fasting, or praying; but the same day that I met him, I went right back to what I knew to do; praying, fasting and reading. I asked myself, "Who is this man?" Little did I know he experienced the same thing, which he shared later on in the courtship. What happened here? Purpose met purpose!!

I decree and declare that The Lord is sending an Elizabeth to help you give birth to your purpose.

Isaiah 66:7-8.
"Before she goes into labor, she gives birth; before the pains come upon her, she delivers a son. Who has ever seen things like this? Can a country be born in a day or a nation be brought forth in a moment? Yet no sooner is Zion in labor than she gives birth to her children."

In Spiritual BIRTH, GOD skips the natural process to bring you deliverance...before your 9 months are up, and before the labor pains start, YOU WILL DELIVER in the first month. Vs 8: "I can turn your life around in one day, I can do things that have never been heard of. Make a nation of people in one day." This is God doing things in our life without the use of natural elements.

I began to meditate on Lamentations 3:21-27. (Message Bible.) You have to find yourself and your situation in the Word of God.

21But there's one other thing I remember, and remembering, I keep a grip on hope:
22-24 God's loyal love couldn't have run out, His merciful love couldn't have dried up.

They're created new every morning.
 How great your faithfulness!
I'm sticking with God (I say it over and over).
 He's all I've got left.
25-27 God proves to be good to the man who passionately waits,
 to the woman who diligently seeks.
It's a good thing to quietly hope,
 quietly hope for help from God.
It's a good thing when you're young
 to stick it out through the hard times.

This is one of my favorite scriptures.

In the midst of pain, sometimes, we really feel that God is not with us, that there is no hope, or He has nothing else for us. But this scripture keeps me reminded that His love and mercies couldn't have run out. There is enough of him to go around. As a matter of fact, His mercies are new every morning.

I'M STICKING WITH GOD. I SAY IT OVER AND OVER AGAIN. HE'S ALL I'VE GOT LEFT. This is a very good place to be. God has proven through all that I have had to encounter. When I could have or should have lost my mind, He was there to keep me.

It's a good thing to quietly hope for help from God.

In the loneliest times, when there is no one around, no one to even share my pain with, those are the times to quietly hope for help from God. There comes a time when we just have to stop talking about to everyone, stop complaining. Go on as if all is well—because it is—and quietly meditate on what He has already done and see it to completion QUIETLY.

CHAPTER 6
THE RELAPSE

Relapse

After the wedding ceremony, we went to the Bahamas for a honeymoon. God is moving and all is well. He's now covering a church in Georgia while we are still living in Florida. We enjoyed traveling back and forth between the two states. Things were great and everyone was happy.

Thirty days into the marriage I noticed things about his attitude I didn't like. The tone of his voice reminded me of my first husband. When he raised his voice at me, I lost it. I mean to the point of cursing him out. I spoke in a language unknown to man. I was furious and I let him have it. I was loud and throwing things around the room. It was truly an explosion in the wrong direction. I never dreamed I could become so angry. I thought I was doing fine until he pushed the wrong buttons. I gave him years of suppressed emotions. I was loud, I was throwing things; it was a total explosion. Now this man is looking at me like, What? I continued and this went on for several days. I continued and I continued. Now remember, this is twenty-three years of hurt that I've never dealt with and what he and I had to realized is that we got married and neither one of us were healed.

Not only did purpose meet purpose, but hurt met hurt. So now he's acting out too. But God is so good—in the midst of both of us acting crazy, saying things we shouldn't say, God begins to deal with us. And what happens when you are not healed is that, whoever you get with the next time, they have to pay for what somebody else did to you before. It's very unfair. I said things to my husband that I can never take back because all my intent was to get him before he got me. I was tired of being on the losing end. So whatever I could conjure up in my spirit or in my head, I said it.

My husband and I both confessed that we brought baggage into the marriage. Our confession led to steps towards healing. If we didn't go through healing, we knew the problems would remain." So we began to meditate on some scriptures and every single day we declared the word of God over our marriage. Every day, we would pray in the spirit and fast together.

As a result, we begin to see a change in each other. I want it to be this way, the right way, all the time, no matter where I am. Righteousness is all the time, not just when I'm at the church. Righteousness should manifest when I'm at home, on my job, and in the mall, and in the grocery store; I have to portray righteousness all the time.

So we had to come up with a prescription that we could take three times a day and we are still doing it. And even at the time of writing this book, the Lord said to me, "Your healing will be complete."

What we have got to understand is you have got to deal with your hurt. Though it has happened to you, you have got to deal with it. There is no way around it; you have got to deal with it. So you have got to figure out, How am I going to deal with this? Because it's going to come out and the very moment that you think you are healed, the trigger comes out and you are going to lose it.

I was speaking with a young lady and she was sharing with me a story about a young lady that she knows that went through some very traumatic events in her life. She was hurt, abused, and so forth, and she ended up marrying someone else after all of this stuff had transpired. And the hurt, because she never dealt with it, she ended up killing her husband and going to prison for fifteen years. Even after getting out of prison, still, the hurt was never dealt with.

Prison is not the answer for hurt. A lot of people are doing things, and they are doing these things because they are not healed and these are triggers. I'm telling you these relapses each time goes to another level. It will only get worst and eventually lead to taking somebody's life. Because, remember I shared with you I didn't even curse when I was in the world and now, all of a sudden, I'm walking in God and I'm cursing my husband. It was because, at the time, it was at another level. Every time, it's going to get worse. So I challenge you to take the time out, starting right now, because even as you are reading, I decree that God is bringing healing to your life right now in Jesus name. But even after reading this book, I challenge you to get a regiment in place that will help you to live, to deal with the hurt.

Be honest about it; we have dressed up for too many years and not going anywhere. We got on the fine clothes, the makeup, the eyelashes, the hair, the weave, but we are not going anywhere. We look good on the outside, but our blood stream is being poisoned from the hurt that we never dealt with. And trust me, it will surface someday. You don't want it to surface to a point where you are going to hurt somebody or take somebody's life. Because this same girl I was talking about, even after fifteen years of her being released, she has been in several relationships, because as soon as she gets in the relationship with these men and that trigger comes, the men are like, "Oh, this lady is crazy or she is demonic." It's not that you're demonic; it's just that you're hurt, and hurting people hurt people. So it's time for your deliverance; it's time for you to be free; it's time for you to deal with this thing called hurt, called pain. We've got to deal with it.

Hurt does not heal itself. If you've ever dealt with anything traumatic, hurtful, or painful, just know it is still there. What we do is go on living life as normal. Eventually, the pain or un-healed hurts will surface and when it does, it is not nice.

Things That Trigger Symptoms

Some people will act out after living through a shocking or dangerous experience. When you're in danger, your body's natural response is to feel scared.

That's when your body turns on its "fight or flight" response. In the face of something life threatening, it revs up your heart rate, sends blood to your muscles to get ready to run, and amps up stress hormones to help fight off bleeding and infection in case you get hurt. Your brain tells your body that some of its functions are less important: Parts of the brain that store memory, emotion, and thinking get "turned off" for a little while.

Normal emotions are shut off from the traumatic experience. That detachment from the memory and the experience can trigger a wrong response after the event.

Traumatic events that are life threatening or related to physical violence or sexual assault can lead to emotional outbreaks:

EXAMPLES

1. Living through a violent act like rape, domestic violence, or sexual, physical, or verbal abuse.
2. Surviving a dangerous event like living through child neglect or abuse.
3. Experiencing the sudden death of a close friend or family member.

In the first month after a severe traumatic event, symptoms similar to PTSD are called an "acute stress disorder" — if those symptoms arise or persist beyond the first month, or develop even years after the event.

Negative response occurs when:

1. Re-experiencing the traumatic event.
2. Experiencing hyper-arousal (muscular and emotional tension).
3. Avoiding situations that may be reminders of the event.
4. Having persistent negative effects on thinking and mood (e.g. emotional numbing).

You will experience:

1. Bad dreams, memories, or flashbacks.
2. Being on edge and easily startled.
3. Feeling emotionally numb and losing interest in things you used to care about.
4. Problems sleeping.
5. Anger and irritability.
6. Hopelessness, depression, thoughts of suicide.
7. Panic attacks.
8. Physical symptoms (headaches, stomach pain, muscle aches, back pain, etc.).

When it comes to relapse or pain, we literally continue with life as normal, as if nothing happened. In the natural, if you cut yourself, after 6 hours, you can no longer get stitches because what you will do is sew up the infection on the inside of the wound, which will in turn filter through the bloodstream poisoning it and later causing sepsis, which will later cause death.

Symptoms of sepsis include either fever or low body temperature, rapid breathing, chills and shaking, rapid heartbeat, decreased urine output, and confusion or delirium.

Sepsis is a life-threatening condition in which the body is fighting a severe infection that has spread via the bloodstream. If a patient becomes "septic," they will likely have low blood pressure leading to poor circulation and lack of blood perfusion of vital tissues and organs. This condition is termed "shock" and is sometimes referred to as septic shock when an infection is the cause of shock to distinguish it from shock due to blood loss or from other causes. This condition can develop either as a result of the body's own defense system or from toxic substances made by the infecting agent. Hospitalized patients are at risk to develop sepsis from infections due to intravenous lines, catheters, surgical wounds, and/or bedsores. The number of people dying from sepsis has increased in the past 20 years. This is most likely due to the increased number of patients who suffer from sepsis.

We have become spiritually septic, causing our bodies to shut down and die because we stitch up our hurt and pain by acting as if we are okay. We try and put all of this church stuff on top of all this pain. Now we are spiritually septic, having poison in our blood stream, and now your death or the death of others will occur.
Let me share a story that was told to me by a co-worker. She had a male

relative who had been married for several years. They had 2 daughters and the dad wanted custody of both girls. Well, the mom said, "You can have the younger one because the 14-year-old is not yours." Can you imagine that? After 14 years of taking care of this child, you find out in an argument concerning divorce that the child is not yours. NOW THAT'S HURT. Well, they divorced and the kids were separated. Years later, he had moved on with his life and so did she. He was in another relationship. Seemed happy. But remember, the hurt was never dealt with. As earlier stated, hurt does not just go away. He was diabetic and called the ex-wife to come and help him because he was not feeling well. She told him no and his next statement was "Okay; well, listen to this" and he pulled the trigger and killed himself. Now that's hurt!!!!!!

Let me help you. Remember, sepsis is the presence of harmful bacteria and their toxins in tissues, typically through infection of a wound.

Septic is a drainage system incorporating a septic tank.

What are you saying, Preacher? I am glad you asked. You have got to figure out a way to drain that hurt out of your system.

Write it out, talk it out. Most of all, be real about what has happened. The more you talk about it, the better it gets.

CHAPTER 7
VICTORY

The song says, "Victory is mine. Victory is mine. Victory today is mine. I told Satan get the behind. Victory today is mine. Hallelujah."

Webster defines victory as the act of defeating an enemy or opponent in a game, battle or competition. For the word of God declares that the battle does not belong to you but the Lord. I realized I had won the victory when I stopped the fight within. When I realized the battle didn't belong to me but God, my victories began to pour in. I saw that my victories sometimes came disguised as defeats; they were unrecognizable in the natural but recognizable in the spirit. I had to learn that in order to receive the victory, I had to push past all the pain. I knew the laboring of my trials would eventually produce the evidence of my delivery

Victory equals a life of peace and joy in the Lord, a life of constant fellowship with the Lord.

A life of victory is a gift. It is a gift offered to us by God, but we must accept it and walk in it. 1Cor 15:57, "Thanks be to God who gives us the victory through our Lord Jesus Christ."

We don't just have victory; we must enter into victory. How? You might ask.

By: (1.) Commit yourself to Christ and (2.) Take Christ as your victory.

We must surrender ourselves, our whole selves to Christ; we must allow Him to order our steps.

Victory is not limited to casting mountains into the sea, or quickly calming turbulent, dangerous situations; victory can also include maintaining an internal attitude of victory during a difficult and prolonged period of time.

Victory is when you can have perseverance in the midst of terrible persecutions, situations.

Victory is the reward of perseverance.

PRAISE gets us and keeps us in victory.

Ex. 15:11, "Who is like unto thee, O Lord, among the gods? Who is like thee, glorious in holiness, fearful in praises, doing wonders?"

* If the scripture says GOD is "Fearful in Praise," that means you need to ENGAGE the power of praise to Provoke the fearful acts of GOD. Whatever is happening in your life that has made everyone around you say, "It would take GOD," can be settled in your Favor by engaging the covenant power of praise, which is your heritage.

Praise is a WEAPON that guarantees Change. Praise is a means through which DIVINE INTERVENTION is Provoked, and divine intervention is the end of Man's FRUSTRATIONS. Praise is the means by which GOD "Takes over your BATTLE."

* No one gets out of the PIT without his hands RAISED UP; and praise is a COVENANT DEVICE with which GOD rescues his people from the "PITS of LIFE."

Ps. 67:5-7, "Let the people PRAISE thee, O GOD; THEN shall the earth YIELD her INCREASE; and GOD, even our OWN GOD, shall Bless us. God shall bless us; and all the ends of the earth shall fear him."

The FEARFUL acts of GOD are PROVOKED by the PRAISES of men.

* If you want to see the "FEARFUL ACTS" of God, then give him a Fearful Dimension of praise. Throw yourself LOOSE in the Praise of his name, Release your DIGNITY, remove your feet from the CHAINS of Hell and Free yourself with the Instrument of PRAISE.

Your PRAISE has the Power to SHAKE loose your PROBLEMS in LIFE.

* Don't be an "OBSERVER" when praise is on. Rather, JOIN others to Praise God, and then will you see his "AMAZING ACTS" in your life.

* King David danced before The Lord with ALL his might, and ALL his mockers were Silenced. Even Michal, his wife that Mocked him, Became BARREN until the day of her DEATH (2 Sam. 6: 14-23).

* Note that Praise has nothing to do with what is happening; rather, it is a CELEBRATION of what is "WRITTEN"!!!!!!!!!!!!!!

Ps. 54:4; 10. "In God I will Praise HIS WORD, in God I have put my Trust; I will not Fear what flesh can do unto me.v10 In God will I Praise his WORD: in The Lord will I praise his word."

PRAISE is different from Thanksgiving:
Thanksgiving- we celebrate what is Happening.
Praise- we celebrate what is WRITTEN.

* And as you Praise him for what is Written, He is Committed to PERFORMING it in your life.

* Praise is a Demonstration of your Faith in GOD!!!! The Lord will PERFECT that which CONCERNS me.

* Therefore, ANYTHING other than good is NOT for you in God's plan. As you give Him praise for these Promises, He will remove ANYTHING in your life that is contrary to them.

The prophet Habakkuk said, "For you to get out of where you are, you MUST give Him the PRAISE that is DUE his nation."

Ps. 22:3, "But thou art Holy; O thou INHABITEST the PRAISES of Israel."

* Praise is the ENVIRONMENT that guarantees DIVINE.

2 chron. 20:22, "And when they BEGIN to SING and to PRAISE, God STEPPED in. They earlier had NO POWER or might against the opposition, but through the Instrument of PRAISE, God set AMBUSHMENT against their enemy."

I decree that EVERY sickness, disease, spell, enchantment, lack of finance working against your DESTINY will be smitten by the Power of PRAISE.

ACTS 16: 25-26, "Paul/Silas prayed and sang PRAISES to God, and God came down at the point where it was 'ABSOLUTELY IMPOSSIBLE' to think of being RESCUED."

* God had no choice but to come down to prove himself. Once the Praises ascends to Heaven, Praise Provokes Divine Presence, which Silences all oppositions and UNFOLDS the path of LIFE.

The Power in Praise:
the Bible's book of 2 Chronicles, chapter 20.

"Word was rushed to Jehoshaphat, the king of Judah, announcing the swift approach of a vast army from Ammon, Moab, and Seir, three kingdoms that had formed an alliance against Judah. Jehoshaphat, knowing that his own army was no match for the invaders, turned to God for help. He proclaimed a time of prayer and fasting, and people from throughout the land poured into the capital to take part.

"Then, in the midst of all the people, Jehoshaphat prayed. 'O Lord, God of our fathers, are You not God in Heaven? You rule over kingdoms and nations, and power and might are in Your hand. None can withstand You.' As the king continued, people's spirits were strengthened. 'We know that in the time of calamity, whatever peril it may be, if we stand in Your presence and cry out to You in our distress, You will hear and save us. We have no power against this great army that comes against us. We do not know what to do, but our eyes are upon You!'

"Then a young priest named Jahaziel prophesied with a loud voice, 'Thus says the Lord to you: "Do not be afraid nor dismayed because of this great multitude, for the battle is not yours, but God's!" God had heard and come to answer their prayers.'

"'You will not need to fight in this battle,' God's message through Jahaziel continued. 'Position yourselves, stand still, and see the salvation of the Lord, who is with you!'

"King Jehoshaphat bowed to the ground in worship. The crowd followed the king's lead, while the priests raised their voices to praise the Lord.

"The next morning as the troops made preparations for battle, King Jehoshaphat encouraged them. 'Believe in the Lord your God, and so shall you be established. Have faith in His prophets, and so shall you have good success.'

"The king consulted with the people, and it was decided that singers should lead the troops into battle. That daring step of faith showed that they believed God would fight for them.

"'Praise the Lord for the beauty of His holiness,' Jehoshaphat instructed the singers as they took their position. 'Give thanks to the Lord, for His mercy endures forever.' They were thanking God in advance for the victory He had promised the day before.

"No sooner had they begun to sing and praise than God 'set ambushes against the people of Ammon, Moab, and Mount Seir, who had come against Judah; and they were defeated.'"

The Bible doesn't specify what those "ambushes" were, but it does explain that the men of those three invading kingdoms began to fight among themselves. First, the men of Ammon and Moab rose up against those of Seir, and when they had destroyed them, the two armies destroyed each other.

"When the army of Judah came to a promontory overlooking the battlefield, they saw only dead bodies on the ground. No one had escaped.

"Jehoshaphat and his men gathered so many valuables from the bodies that it took them three days to collect them all.

"On the fourth day they assembled in the Valley of Berachah, which means 'the Valley of Praise,' and there they blessed God. Then they returned home with joy, for the Lord had triumphed over their enemies.

"The fear of God came on all the neighboring kingdoms when they heard how He had interceded for Judah, and 'the realm of Jehoshaphat was quiet, for his God gave him rest all around.'"

What an amazing testimony to the power of faith, prayer, and praise—and that same power is available to us today. Whenever we face problems, pain, hurt that is too big for us, if we pray with our whole hearts and believe the promises God has given us in His Word, we can then go on the attack against whatever it is that threatens to undo us, praising the Lord and thanking Him by faith for the victory, and He will bring us the victory.

I feel really good about this victory; this new place in God. Tamela man sings a song titled "THIS PLACE" that I just love to listen to.

In this place that I never knew, never even imagined is really real. This is a place where I am free for real. A place where I am experiencing God like I never have before.

In this new season, I am writing books, I am mentoring women who are seeking kingdom experiences, I am working on my bachelors in theology, I am traveling in ministry preaching the Gospel of JESUS. I can now relate to those that are broken, suicidal and dismayed. I am hearing and seeing spiritually like never before. I am co- pastor with my husband who teaches me daily the Word of God. This is my Victory. I can truly say that the pain was worth it. The pain pushed me, or should I say, thrust me to my destiny. You see, without pain, there is no birthing. NO PAIN, NO BIRTHING.

Majority of women desires giving birth to a child. Even as a child, when asked what we wanted to do when we grow up, most of us would say, "I wanted to get married, have 2 children, a dog, and a white picket fence."

In the desires, we never focus on the pain that we will have to go through together, that we've dreamed about. Well, there is a pain that comes with giving birth.

There are some things that we are even believing God for pertaining to our purpose or destiny. We are focusing on the good things that come with destiny when in reality we will go through the birthing pains first in order to give birth to our destiny.

Well, in a nutshell, I am writing to you totally victorious; nothing missing, nothing broken. I am whole, complete, and entire. My victory came when I realized that there was something worthwhile on the other side of pain.

If you can muster up enough strength in the midst of your pain to mentally turn that thing over, then that's where you will find your purpose, your peace, your deliverance, your healing, and your breakthrough.

See, the enemy wants you to think that pain is all you get or deserve. But, my sisters and brothers, I beg to differ. God has given everything pertaining to life and Godliness. Grab it. It's on the other side of the pain.

The Bible declares Jacob wrestled with the angel all night. He was determined not let go until he was blessed by him.

God is calling for someone that will hang in there, and don't let go—even if you have to leave with a Limp. It's just a reminder that you are in it to win it.
I may be limping, I may still have pain but because the Bible declares that I am victorious, then it's just that.

I WIN!!!!!

I am at the end of this book, but the beginning of my new life. I am learning in the midst of every situation just to find myself or my situation in the word and stand on it. See, God is only obligated to his word. He said that his word will nerve fail.

You can cry, scream, throw tantrum; that does not move God. He is only obligated to his word.

In victory, it does not mean that pain will never show up. It means when it does, I now know how to flip it over and keep moving in the things of God.

Until the Ancient of days came—Notes, Daniel 7:9. That is, this was to occur after the horn grew to its full size, and after the war was made with the saints, and they had been overcome. It does not affirm that this would occur immediately, but that at some subsequent period the Ancient of days would come, and would set up a kingdom on the earth, or would make over the kingdom to the saints. There would be as real a transfer and as actual a setting up of a peculiar kingdom, as if God Himself should appear on the earth, and should publicly make over the dominion to them.

And judgment was given to the saints of the Most High—that is, there was a solemn act of judgement in the case by which the kingdom was given to their hands. It was as real a transfer as if there had been a judgment pronounced on the beast, and he had been condemned and overthrown, and as if the dominion which he once had should be made over to the servants of the Most High.

And the time came that the saints possessed the kingdom—that they ruled on the earth; that good men made and administered the laws; that the principles of religion prevailed, influencing the hearts of all men, and causing righteousness and justice to be done. The universal prevalence of true religion, in controlling the hearts and lives of men, and disposing them to do what in all circumstances ought to be done, would be a complete fulfillment of all that is here said. Thus far the description of what Daniel saw, of which he was so desirous to obtain an explanation. The explanation follows and embraces the remainder of the chapter. It looked like, felt like hurt and pain was winning. I even felt defeated. But God, The spirit of God showed up and declared victory over the pain, the hurt, the defeat. See, the enemy wants you to think and believe that it is over. But how many of you know that the devil is a liar and the father of lies? My sisters and my brothers, I decree and declare that the Lord Himself has declared favor over your situation, over your restoration in JESUS NAME. GUESS WHAT? WE WIN!

In order to have victory, you must have determination. You must change the way you think. You must not think in your situation, but think outside of your situation; seeing yourself in the winner's circle. You must speak victory until you see victory. Remember the little engine that could; as long as he looked at that mountain as too big for him to climb, he didn't climb but when he changed how he saw the mountain and himself, he started to believe he could do it. It started with, I think I can and after while he started saying, "I know I can," and he made it up to the top. He changed his way of thinking.

There is testimony that I have to share. In 2011, God manifested His Divine Healing to me. Let me start from the beginning. For several months, I was very weak and tired. I noticed that as I walked up my stairs, I would begin to have heart palpitations and I would literally have to lay and rest before I could go back down the stairs. I knew something was wrong but in all honesty, I was afraid to go to the doctor. After several months, I grew worse. Finally, one day as I walked into my garage, I began to feel very light-headed, dizzy, I felt very hot and then collapsed to the floor. My husband took me to the doctor's office and there in the waiting area I passed out again. The doctor picked me up off the floor and carried me to the back. After examining me, he said that my nail beds were white, there was no pink color to my fingertips. He said to me, "You do not have any blood; you need to go to the hospital immediately for blood transfusion." Wow, it was very scary and all I could think in my mind was "I should have gone to the doctor when I first started having symptoms." Well, now I am admitted to the hospital. They began to draw blood to see just where my levels were. My internal medicine doctor came in with the result and my hemoglobin was 4. The normal range for an adult woman is 12–16. My platelet count was 99,000. The normal range for an adult is 150,000-450,000. My levels were way too low. The doctor was very concerned. He could not understand how I was still functioning. They started the blood transfusions. After checking my levels again the next morning, my levels were still the same. My doctor had now contacted the oncologist (cancer specialist/hematologist) and OB/GYN. They are trying figure out why I was bleeding out or where was I bleeding from. Ok, now I am really scared. You know it is something about the C word that puts your mind in another area. I was given 2 more pints of blood. On day 4 in the hospital, things were getting worse; levels were declining. My hemoglobin was still at 4 but the platelet count had dropped to 30,000 from 99,000. So this was serious. The doctor explained that there was not much he could do. He said that I should not go to the bathroom or walk alone. I said to him, "Listen, I feel fine; just give me another pint of blood so that I can go home." He looked at my husband and said, "This does not look good, she is bleeding out. Her body is destroying the blood from the transfusion, so there is no need of transfusing her anymore. She will probably not make it through the night." At this point, I began to cry and call on the God that I had been serving faithfully. I said, "My God, I don't believe that I have completed my assignment in the earth. There is still more that I need to minister to. My purpose cannot be complete." My husband called all the family and they all came to see me. My brother began to pray and declare the Word of God over my situation. At that point, I really received the Word of God that was released and I commanded my body to come into alignment with the word of God. The next day the doctor came in the room to see me. The nurse had come by earlier that morning to draw blood. The doctor then told me that my platelet count was even lower; at 9,000 at the time. I didn't panic over this because I had totally given it all to God and I was believing without wavering that he was going to do it! Again, he said that there was nothing he could do and left the room. How many of you know that when the doctors have done all they could do, it is a good place for God? Man's extremities are God's opportunities.

I believed that supernaturally, God was going to do something. The next morning, the nurse came into my room to draw blood to check my levels. Of course they could not understand how I was feeling so well and were still in awe that I was still alive. Well, here we go. Look at the hand of God. The cancer specialist came into my room and said, "Something happened last night. Your platelet count has increased from 9,000 to 100,000 but we will keep you another day because your body is fighting against itself so it will probably change." My exact words to her was: "NO NO NO, my God doesn't halfway do anything; if He started it, He will finish it." Well, here we are on the next day—Saturday. The doctor came back in with results from the early morning blood draw. She said, "This has to be God because your hemoglobin is now at 12, which is normal, and your platelet count has increased to 160,000." Wow! Excuse me for about 30 seconds to give God a shout. He is worthy to be praised. I left the hospital that day knowing that MY GOD is truly a HEALER. By the way, all of the tests that they did were all normal.

Now that's VICTORY!!

CONCLUSION

In the Bible, Paul declares, "Three times I pleaded with the Lord to take it away from me. 9 But he said to me, 'My grace is sufficient for you, for my power is made perfect in weakness.' Therefore I will boast all the more gladly about my weaknesses, so that Christ's power may rest on me."

Pain is inevitable. Pain comes and goes. As you can see in scripture with Paul, that which represented pain in his life never left. So, what do we do about this thing called pain? I am so glad that you asked.

JUST FLIP IT OVER. In order to see what's on the other side of pain, we've got to simply flip it over to see what's on the other side. Why wait until the pain have ended? Go ahead now to get a sneak preview of the awesome experience that awaits just on the other side.

I need you to stop for a moment, sit still and mentally see you outside of pain. That's where your purpose is hiding.

You just have to come to realize like I did in my promiscuity, the abuse, the low self-esteem, the depression, that there has to be more.

I had to begin to decree some things over my own life. I KNOW GOD DID NOT CREATE ME FOR THIS MESS THAT I AM IN. THERE HAS TO BE MORE TO MY BEING CREATED THAN THIS. I was very angry at myself and my situation because I knew that there was more. I've come to realize that until we get sick and tired of being sick and tired, we will remain the same. You've got to get mad and take your purpose.

It's not far; just on the other side of the pain. On the other side, there is greatness, there is power, there is wealth, success, and abundance.

Stop focusing on what you have gone through and what you are going through and just that you have a purpose. Just change your thinking. We have to understand that pain will come and sometimes it won't leave. My sisters and my brothers, be encouraged because God will never leave you or forsake you and He is with you even until the end of the world. We have to literally turn pain to the other side. What if it doesn't leave? Are you going to just sit there in pity and abort your purpose? No! You will look on the other side of the pain because that's where your peace is. That's where your purpose is. That's where your destiny lies. That's where your deliverance is. That's where your joy is. I know you think that it's over. I know that you have almost given up. No, the best is yet to come. You had to go through that to get to this. I am shouting, "FLIP OVER PAIN. JUST TURN IT OVER!!!!" See what's on the other side of PAIN.

PRAYER DECREES

Thou shalt also decree a thing, and it shall be established unto thee; and the light shall shine upon thine ways (Job 22:28).

"I" or "WE" DECREE:

1. Today marks the END of every oppression that the devil has placed on my life.
2. I am an overcomer!
3. Every seemingly UNCROSSABLE BARRIER of my life, by the two wings of a great eagle, will cause me this day to FLY over all of my barriers.
4. Every force that is pressing hard against my DESTINY will not escape and shall be drowned in the Spiritual Red Sea.
5. I am moving in the NEXT PHASE OF MY DESTINY.
6. Every sickness, disease, spell, enchantment, lack of finance working against my destiny will be smitten by the Power of Praise
7. The Spirit of God will enter me and empower me into the next level.
8. My past will no longer hinder my present or future.
9. Through prayer there will be an outbreak of Power demonstrated all around me TODAY!
10. The Light will turn on in my heart to make darkness flee!
11. An ERUPTION is taking place in my life right NOW!
12. EVERYTHING that has kept me down, in the Name of Jesus Christ, I am walking out of them!
13. ANY force that is sitting on my DESTINY today must bow down in the Name of Jesus!

14. TODAY is my day of LIBERTY!
15. I am strengthened to overcome and reign with Jesus.
16. My mind is being restored!!
17. The years the locust, the palmerworms, and the cankerworms have eaten will now be restored!
18. God's glorious presence will be visibly seen in my life.
19. The awesome, weighty presence of God will become heavier and heavier!
20. He who has begun a good work in me WILL complete it.
21. Angels who are present-time ministers are connecting me to destiny assignments. They are protecting my purpose. They are wrestling DESTINY out for me.
22. I will have success, prosperity, and financial security.
23. The same God who opened a Promised Land for Moses and the Israelites is doing it for you. Places of promise are opening to me NOW!
24. I declare my FREEDOM today!
25. The windows of heaven are open over me, according to The Word of God.
26. The blessings of God will overtake me.
27. Decide NOW to make your life grander, greater, richer, and noble than ever before.
28. I now sow thoughts of peace, happiness, right action, goodwill, and prosperity.
29. I am beautiful, strong and powerful.
30. I am God's gift to this world.
31. There is a king in me.
32. I am victorious!
33. It's my time and season to do what God has called me to do.
34. RECEIVE a fresh Spirit of BOLDNESS on your new life NOW!

ENDNOTES

1. David Oyedepo , http://pulse.ng/religion/david-oyedepo-udom-s-victory-is-the-triumph-of-light-over-darkness-id4674200.html; accessed November 02, 2016.

2. Tim Sheets, Angel Armies (Shippensburg, PA: DESTINY IMAGE PUBLISHERS INC.,2016)

3. Myles Munroe, quoted on http://paulsohn.org/top-15-myles-munroe-quotes-of-all-time/; accessed November 10, 2014

4. Steve Pavlina, http://www.stevepavlina.com/blog/2005/01/how-to-discover-your-life-purpose-in-about-20-minutes/ ;accessed January 16, 2005

ABOUT THE AUTHOR

Pastor Vicki Head Jackson is a native of Jackson, Ga. Born to the parents of Benjamin and Virginia Head. She is the Executive Pastor of Kingdom Living Ministries. Atlanta, Ga. Attended Gordon College in Barnesville, Ga, with an Associates in General Studies. In 1998, she graduated from Advanced Career Training Medical Institute and has been working in the medical field for 20 years. She is now attending Andersonville Theological Seminary to obtain her bachelor degree in theology. She is married to Gerald Jackson and together, they have 3 sons. She is an author, writer, psalmist, worship leader, and teacher. She is the founder of Women of Purpose—a Women's Ministry. Her call of God is to help the hurting women, liberating, and empowering them to walk in their God-ordained purpose without reservation.

MINISTRY CONTACT INFORMATION:
Vicki Head Jackson

678-371-6470

Made in the USA
Charleston, SC
16 December 2016